SJOGREN'S SYNDROME DIET RECIPES COOKBOOK

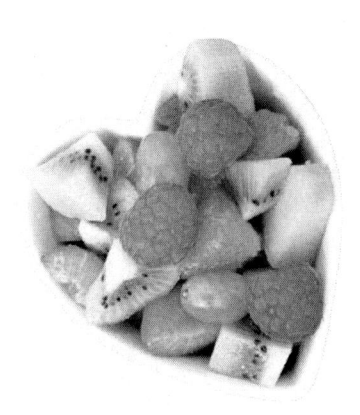

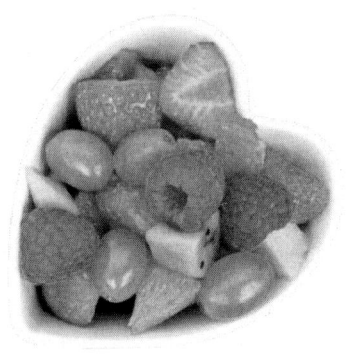

DR. PENNY WATSON

Copyright © 2023 by Dr. Penny Watson

All rights reserved. No part of this publication may be reproduced, distributed, or transmitted in any form or by any means, including photocopying, recording, or other electronic or mechanical methods, without the prior written permission of the publisher, except in the case of brief quotations embodied in critical reviews and certain other noncommercial uses permitted by copyright law.

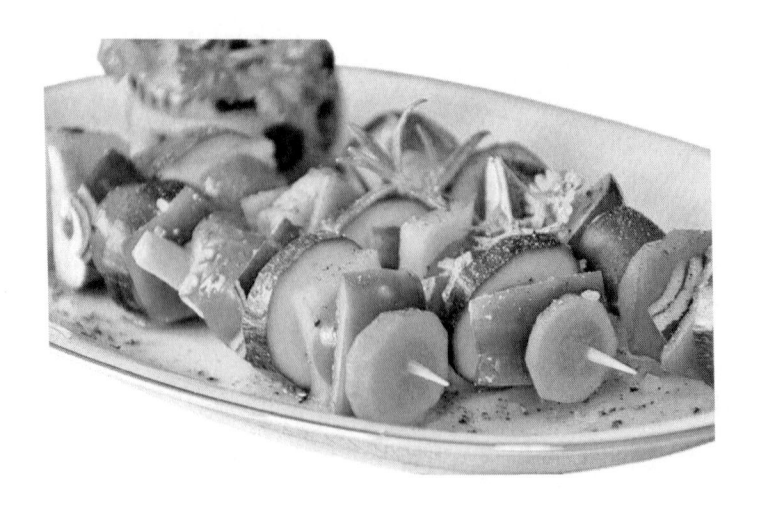

Table of Contents

INTRODUCTION 7

CHAPTER ONE 11

  Sjogren's Syndrome Explained....................... 11

  Types Of Sjogren's Syndrome........................ 13

  Causes Of Sjogren's Syndrome 14

  Viral And Bacterial Infection as a Cause for Sjogren's Syndrome 15

  Symptoms Of Sjogren's Syndrome 17

CHAPTER TWO 19

  Sjogren's Syndrome Diets and Benefits 19

  How To Follow Sjogren's Syndrome Diet 21

  Foods to Avoid... 22

  Foods to Include.. 22

  Tips for Following a Sjogren's Syndrome Diet............ 23

  7-Day Sjogren's Syndrome Meal Plan 24

Day 1 24

Day 2 28

Day 3 31

Day 4 34

Day 5 37

Day 6 41

Day 7 43

CHAPTER THREE 49

Sjogren's Syndrome Recipes 49

BREAKFAST 49

1. Banana Pancakes with Honey 49

2. Yogurt Parfait with Berries 50

3. Avocado Toast with Eggs 50

4. Oatmeal with Nuts and Dates 51

5. Poached Pears with Ricotta 52

6. Egg and Cheese Sandwich 53

7. Smoothie Bowl with Berries 54

8. Omelette with Spinach 54

9. Greek Yogurt with Nuts and Honey 55

10. Fruit and Nut Granola Bars 56

11. Salmon and Asparagus with Garlic Lemon Sauce .. 56

12. Vegetable and Quinoa Stew 58

13. Creamy Cauliflower Soup 59

14. Avocado and Tomato Quinoa Salad 61

15. Baked Cod with Spinach and Tomatoes 62

16. No-Bake Oatmeal Cookies 63

17. Zucchini and Carrot Fritters 64

18. Baked Sweet Potato Fries 65

19. Baked Eggplant Parmesan 66

20. Banana Oat Smoothie 68

LUNCH 69

1. Salmon and Avocado Wraps 69

2. Quinoa and Vegetable Bowl 70

3. Sesame Chicken Salad 71

4. Salmon and Broccoli Bowl 72

5. Zucchini and Tomato Salad 73

6. Sweet Potato and Bean Burrito 74

7. Avocado and Egg Salad 75

8. Grilled Vegetable Wrap 76

9. Lentil and Spinach Salad – 20 minutes 77

10. Mushroom and Quinoa Bowl – 25 minutes 78

DINNER 79

1. Spanish-Style Stuffed Peppers 79

2. Baked Salmon with Roasted Vegetables 81

3. Quinoa Bowl with Turkey and Veggies 82

4. Slow Cooker Chicken and Quinoa Stew 83

5. Sautéed Shrimp and Veggies 84

CONCLUSION 87

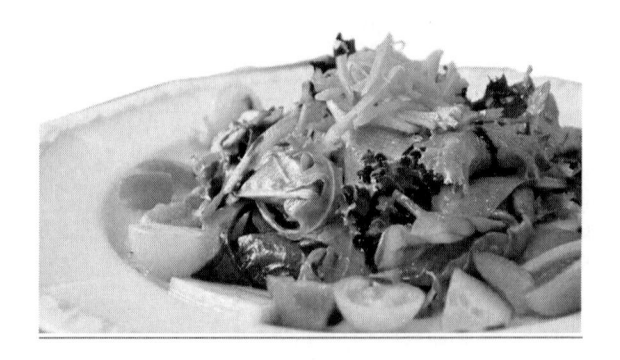

INTRODUCTION

Once upon a time there was a young woman named Sarah. She was a passionate chef who dreamed of one day writing a cookbook of her own.

One day, Sarah heard about a rare medical condition called Sjogren's Syndrome. People with this condition often experience dry eyes, dry mouth and extreme fatigue. She was moved by the plight of those suffering from this condition and wanted to do something to help.

Sarah decided to dedicate her cooking skills to creating a cookbook filled with recipes that could help those with Sjogren's Syndrome. She took her time to research and develop recipes that would provide the right combination of nutrition and flavor. Focusing on ingredients such as omega-3 fatty acids, zinc, and magnesium, Sarah created a variety of delicious meals and snacks to help those with Sjogren's Syndrome manage their symptoms.

After months of hard work, Sarah's cookbook was published. It was met with an overwhelmingly positive response from the Sjogren's Syndrome community.

People wrote in to thank Sarah for her dedication to helping them eat well and manage their symptoms.

Thanks to Sarah's hard work, Sjogren's Syndrome sufferers now have access to a cookbook filled with recipes that provide the right combination of nutrition and flavor. She proved that with the right diet, Sjogren's syndrome sufferers can lead healthier lives.

Sjogren's syndrome is a chronic autoimmune disorder that affects the body's moisture-producing glands. It is one of the most common autoimmune disorders, affecting approximately 3 million people in the United States alone. Symptoms of Sjogren's syndrome can include dry eyes, dry mouth, fatigue, and joint pain.

In some cases, people with Sjogren's syndrome may also experience more serious symptoms, such as kidney disease, lung disease, and nerve damage. While there is no cure for Sjogren's syndrome, treatments such as medications, lifestyle modifications, and alternative therapies can help manage the symptoms.

Sjogren's syndrome is an autoimmune disorder, which means that it is caused by a malfunction of the immune system. Normally, the immune system is responsible for defending the body against germs and other foreign invaders.

In people with Sjogren's syndrome, the immune system mistakenly attacks the body's own moisture-producing glands, including those in the eyes and mouth. This causes the glands to become inflamed and unable to produce enough moisture.

The exact cause of Sjogren's syndrome is unknown, but it is believed to be a combination of genetic and environmental factors. People with certain genetic markers have a higher risk of developing the disorder. Additionally, certain environmental triggers, such as certain medications, infections, or stress, may increase the risk.

Sjogren's syndrome can be difficult to diagnose, as the symptoms can be similar to those of other conditions. Additionally, some people with Sjogren's syndrome may not experience any symptoms, making diagnosis even more difficult.

To diagnose the condition, doctors will typically perform a physical exam, ask the patient about their medical history, and order lab tests to check for the presence of specific antibodies.

Although there is no cure for Sjogren's syndrome, there are treatments available to help manage the symptoms. Medications, such as nonsteroidal anti-inflammatory drugs (NSAIDs), corticosteroids, and immunosuppressants, can help reduce inflammation and relieve pain.

Additionally, lifestyle modifications, such as avoiding spicy or acidic foods, drinking plenty of fluids, and wearing sunglasses when outdoors, can help reduce dryness and irritation.

Alternative therapies, such as acupuncture, massage therapy, and hypnosis, may also be helpful in managing symptoms.

Sjogren's syndrome is a chronic condition that can have a significant impact on a person's quality of life. While there is no cure, treatments can help manage the symptoms and improve a person's comfort and well-being.

With proper treatment and lifestyle modifications, people with Sjogren's syndrome can still lead active, fulfilling lives.

CHAPTER ONE

Sjogren's Syndrome Explained

Sjogren's syndrome is an autoimmune disorder that causes dryness in the eyes, mouth, and other parts of the body. The disorder is named after the Swedish physician, Henrik Sjogren, who first described it in 1933. For people with Sjogren's, it can be difficult to find the right diet to help manage their symptoms.

Nutrition is an important part of managing Sjogren's syndrome. A balanced diet can help minimize symptoms and prevent the development of complications. People with Sjogren's should focus on eating a variety of healthy foods, such as lean proteins, whole grains, fruits, and vegetables. Additionally, it's important to stay hydrated and drink plenty of water throughout the day.

It's important to note that there is no one-size-fits-all diet for people with Sjogren's syndrome. Everyone's dietary needs are different, and it's important to work with a dietitian to find the best plan for you.

Some general tips for those with Sjogren's include eating smaller meals more frequently throughout the day, avoiding spicy and acidic foods that can trigger symptoms, and limiting caffeine and sugar intake. Additionally, eating foods that are high in fibre, such as fruits, vegetables, and whole grains, is beneficial for overall digestive health.

It's also important to pay attention to food sensitivities. Some people with Sjogren's may be sensitive to certain ingredients, such as dairy, gluten, or certain preservatives. Paying attention to any food sensitivities and avoiding those foods can help reduce symptoms.

Finally, it's important to pay attention to your individual needs and listen to your body. If certain foods seem to trigger symptoms, it's important to avoid them. Additionally, it's important to practice mindful eating and maintain a healthy weight.

Overall, eating a healthy, balanced diet is important for managing Sjogren's syndrome. It's important to work with a dietitian to find the best plan for you.

Additionally, it's important to pay attention to food sensitivities and practice mindful eating.

With the right diet and lifestyle changes, it is possible to manage Sjogren's syndrome and reduce symptoms.

Types Of Sjogren's Syndrome

Sjogren's syndrome is an autoimmune disorder characterized by the dryness of the eyes, mouth, and other areas of the body. It is caused by the body's immune system attacking its own moisture-producing glands. There are three main types of Sjogren's syndrome: primary, secondary, and Sicca syndrome.

1. Primary Sjogren's Syndrome: This type of Sjogren's is the most common. It affects the tear and saliva glands, resulting in dry eyes and dry mouth. It might also induce weariness and joint discomfort

2. Secondary Sjogren's Syndrome: This type of Sjogren's is caused by another underlying autoimmune disorder. It is associated with conditions such as lupus, rheumatoid arthritis, and scleroderma. It can cause the same symptoms as primary Sjogren's Syndrome.

3. Sicca Syndrome: Sicca Syndrome is characterized by dry eyes and dry mouth, but without any other signs of Sjogren's Syndrome.

It is often associated with other autoimmune disorders such as rheumatoid arthritis and lupus.

4. Subclinical Sjogren's Syndrome: This type of Sjogren's is characterized by dry eyes and dry mouth but without any other symptoms. It is often difficult to diagnose and is considered a mild form of the disease.

5. Neonatal Sjogren's Syndrome: This type of Sjogren's is very rare and affects newborn babies. It is characterized by inflammation of the glands that produce tears and saliva, leading to dry eyes and dry mouth.

Causes Of Sjogren's Syndrome

Sjogren's Syndrome is an autoimmune disorder characterized by inflammation of the tear and saliva glands, leading to dry eyes and dry mouth. The exact cause of Sjogren's Syndrome is unknown, but there are a number of factors that may contribute to its development.

1. Genetics: Sjogren's Syndrome may have a genetic component as it has been found to run in families.

2. Gender: Women are more likely to develop Sjogren's Syndrome than men.

3. Age: Sjogren's Syndrome typically affects people over the age of 40.

4. Viral and Bacterial Infections: Certain viral and bacterial infections have been linked to the development of Sjogren's Syndrome, such as hepatitis C and the Epstein-Barr virus.

5. Autoimmune Conditions: People with other autoimmune conditions, such as rheumatoid arthritis and systemic lupus erythematosus, are more likely to develop Sjogren's Syndrome.

6. Stress: Stress can trigger the autoimmune response that leads to the symptoms of Sjogren's Syndrome.

7. Smoking: Research has found that smoking may increase the risk of developing Sjogren's Syndrome.

Viral And Bacterial Infection as a Cause for Sjogren's Syndrome

Sjogren's Syndrome is an autoimmune disorder that affects the body's ability to produce moisture, including tears and saliva. It is characterized by dry eyes and a dry mouth, among other symptoms.

While there is no known cause for the condition, research suggests that viral and bacterial infections may play a role in its development.

Viral infections, such as Epstein-Barr virus (EBV) and Cytomegalovirus (CMV), have been linked to the development of Sjogren's Syndrome.

EBV is the virus that causes mononucleosis, and it is believed that it can trigger the immune system to attack the glands responsible for producing moisture.

CMV is a common virus that is present in most people, and it is thought that an overactive immune system may cause it to attack the glands as well.

Bacterial infections, such as Mycoplasma pneumoniae and Chlamydia pneumoniae, have also been linked to Sjogren's Syndrome.

Mycoplasma pneumoniae is a type of bacteria that causes respiratory illnesses, and it is believed that this bacterium can trigger the immune system to attack the glands responsible for producing moisture.

Chlamydia pneumoniae, on the other hand, is a type of bacteria that causes genital infections, and it is believed that it can also trigger an overactive immune system.

In some cases, researchers believe that a combination of viral and bacterial infections can lead to the development of Sjogren's Syndrome.

For example, if a person has an active EBV infection, and then contracts a bacterial infection such as Mycoplasma pneumoniae or Chlamydia pneumoniae, this may cause the immune system to become overactive and attack the glands responsible for producing moisture.

The exact cause of Sjogren's Syndrome is still unknown, but viral and bacterial infections appear to be linked to the condition. While there is no cure for the condition, treatments are available to help manage its symptoms.

Symptoms Of Sjogren's Syndrome

Sjogren's syndrome is an autoimmune disorder which affects the body's ability to produce moisture. It can cause a variety of symptoms, which generally fall into two categories:

1. Dryness Symptoms: Dry eyes, dry mouth, dry skin, dry nose, dry throat, dry vagina, dry cough, and dry lips.

2. Inflammation Symptoms: Joint pain, fatigue, rashes, and inflammation of the major salivary glands.

3. Other Symptoms: Difficulty speaking and swallowing, swollen lymph nodes, and recurrent infections.

4. Systemic Symptoms: Neurological problems, depression, and an increased risk of developing certain cancers.

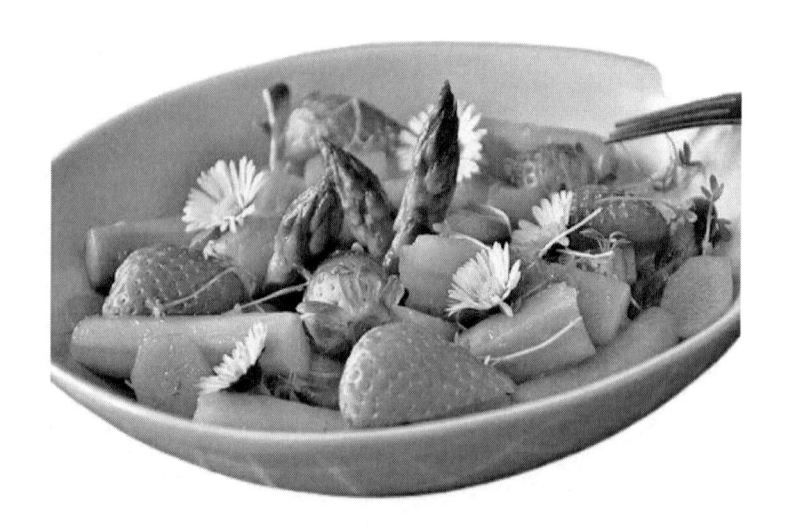

CHAPTER TWO

Sjogren's Syndrome Diets and Benefits

Sjogren's syndrome is an autoimmune disorder that affects the salivary and tear glands, leading to dry eyes and dry mouth. It is important for those with Sjogren's syndrome to eat a healthy, balanced diet to help manage their symptoms and minimize the risk of developing other health problems.

The most important dietary recommendation for those with Sjogren's syndrome is to stay well hydrated. This is especially important for those who have dry eyes and dry mouth.

Drinking plenty of fluids throughout the day can help reduce the discomfort associated with these symptoms. Additionally, staying hydrated can help prevent constipation, which is a common symptom of Sjogren's syndrome.

In addition to staying hydrated, it is important to consume a balanced diet that is high in fibre, vitamins, and minerals.

Whole grains, fruits, and vegetables are all excellent sources of fibre, vitamins, and minerals and should be included in the diet.

Additionally, lean proteins such as fish, poultry, and beans can help provide the body with the nutrients it needs to stay healthy.

Those with Sjogren's syndrome should also be mindful of the types and amounts of fats they consume. It is important to limit saturated fats, trans fats, and cholesterol, and instead opt for healthier unsaturated fats such as those found in nuts and avocados.

Additionally, it is important to avoid added sugars and processed foods, as these can contribute to inflammation and other health problems.

It is also important to pay attention to food intolerances and allergies. Many people with Sjogren's syndrome have difficulty digesting certain foods, which can lead to uncomfortable symptoms. Paying attention to any adverse reactions to food can help identify any food intolerances and allergies.

Eating a healthy, balanced diet is important for everyone, but it is especially important for those with Sjogren's syndrome. Eating a balanced diet can help manage symptoms, reduce the risk of other health problems, and ensure that the body receives all of the nutrients it needs to stay healthy. Additionally, it is important to pay attention to food intolerances and allergies and stay well hydrated to help manage symptoms and prevent other health problems.

By eating a healthy, balanced diet and paying attention to food intolerances and allergies, those with Sjogren's syndrome can help ensure that their overall health and quality of life is maintained.

How To Follow Sjogren's Syndrome Diet

Sjogren's syndrome is an autoimmune disorder that causes dryness in the body, most commonly in the eyes, mouth and nose.

It can also affect the skin, joints, and other organs. Following a Sjogren's syndrome diet can help manage the symptoms of this chronic condition.

This article will discuss the foods to avoid, the foods to include, and tips for following a Sjogren's syndrome diet.

Foods to Avoid:

• **Processed and refined sugars:** Foods high in sugar can cause inflammation in the body and should be avoided.

• **Salt:** High salt intake can lead to dehydration which can worsen symptoms of Sjogren's syndrome.

• **Caffeine:** Caffeine can interfere with hydration and exacerbate symptoms.

• **Dairy:** Dairy products can increase mucous production and should be avoided.

• **Gluten:** Gluten can trigger an autoimmune response and should be avoided.

• **Alcohol:** Alcohol can cause dehydration and worsen symptoms.

Foods to Include:

• **Fruits and Vegetables:** Eating plenty of fruits and vegetables can provide the body with necessary vitamins and minerals.

- **High-fibre Foods:** Eating high-fibre foods can help keep the digestive system running smoothly.

- **Omega-3 Rich Foods:** Omega-3 fatty acids can help reduce inflammation in the body.

- **Healthy Fats:** Eating healthy fats such as olive oil, nuts and seeds can provide the body with essential fatty acids.

- **Lean Proteins:** Eating lean proteins such as fish, chicken and eggs can help provide the body with essential amino acids.

Tips for Following a Sjogren's Syndrome Diet

- **Stay Hydrated:** Staying hydrated is essential for managing Sjogren's syndrome.

- **Eat Smaller Meals:** Eating smaller meals throughout the day can help keep the digestive system running smoothly.

- **Avoid Trigger Foods:** Avoiding foods that can trigger an autoimmune response can help reduce symptoms.

- **Get Enough Sleep:** Getting enough sleep can help the body recover and reduce inflammation.

- **Exercise Regularly:** Exercise can help reduce inflammation and improve overall health.

Following a Sjogren's syndrome diet can help manage the symptoms of this chronic condition. Eating plenty of fruits and vegetables, high-fibre foods, omega-3 rich foods, healthy fats, and lean proteins can help reduce inflammation and improve overall health.

Avoiding processed and refined sugars, salt, caffeine, dairy, gluten and alcohol can also help reduce symptoms. Staying hydrated, eating smaller meals, avoiding trigger foods, getting enough sleep, and exercising regularly can also help manage Sjogren's syndrome.

7-Day Sjogren's Syndrome Meal Plan

Day 1

Breakfast:

Overnight Oatmeal

Ingredients:

-1/2 cup rolled oats

-1/3 cup plain Greek yogurt

-1/2 cup almond milk

-1 teaspoon flaxseed

-1/2 teaspoon ground cinnamon

-1/4 teaspoon vanilla extract

-1 teaspoon honey.

Instructions:

In a medium bowl, combine oats, yogurt, almond milk, flaxseed, cinnamon, and vanilla extract. Refrigerate the bowl overnight, covered. In the morning, top with honey and enjoy.

Lunch:

Roasted Vegetable Salad:

Ingredients:

-1 cup diced sweet potato

-1/2 cup red bell pepper, diced

-1/2 cup yellow bell pepper, diced

-1/2 cup red onion, diced

-1 tablespoon olive oil

-1/4 teaspoon garlic powder

-1/4 teaspoon black pepper

-1/4 teaspoon salt

-2 cups arugula

-1/4 cup feta cheese

-2 tablespoons balsamic vinegar

Instructions:

Preheat oven to 400 degrees F. Line a baking sheet with parchment paper. In a medium bowl, combine sweet potato, bell peppers, red onion, olive oil, garlic powder, black pepper, and salt.

Spread mixture on the prepared baking sheet and roast for 20-25 minutes, stirring halfway through. In a large bowl, combine roasted vegetables and arugula.

Top with feta cheese and balsamic vinegar. Serve.

Dinner:

Baked Salmon with Garlic-Lemon Sauce:

Ingredients:

-2 salmon fillets

-2 teaspoons olive oil

-1/4 teaspoon garlic powder

-1/4 teaspoon black pepper

-1/4 teaspoon salt

-1/4 cup white wine

-3 tablespoons lemon juice

-2 tablespoons butter

Instructions:

Preheat oven to 375 degrees F. Line a baking sheet with parchment paper.

Place salmon fillets on the prepared baking sheet and brush with olive oil.

Season with garlic powder, black pepper, and salt. Roast for 15-20 minutes, or until salmon is cooked through.

Meanwhile, in a small saucepan over medium heat, combine white wine, lemon juice, and butter.

Cook for 3-4 minutes, or until the sauce thickens. Serve salmon with garlic-lemon sauce.

Day 2

Breakfast:

Blueberry Chia

Ingredients:

-1/2 cup plain Greek yogurt

-1/2 cup almond milk

-1 tablespoon chia seeds

-1/2 teaspoon ground cinnamon

-1/4 teaspoon vanilla extract

-1/2 cup fresh blueberries

-1 teaspoon honey

Instructions:

In a medium bowl, combine yogurt, almond milk, chia seeds, cinnamon, and vanilla extract.

Place the bowl in the refrigerator overnight.

In the morning, top with blueberries and honey. Enjoy.

Lunch:

Salmon and Avocado Sandwich:

Ingredients:

-2 slices whole-wheat bread

-1 salmon fillet, cooked and flaked

-1/4 avocado, mashed

-2 teaspoons olive oil

-1 teaspoon lemon juice

-1/4 teaspoon garlic powder

-1/4 teaspoon black pepper

-1/4 teaspoon salt

-1/4 cup arugula

Instructions:

In a small bowl, combine mashed avocado, olive oil, lemon juice, garlic powder, black pepper, and salt.

Spread mixture on one slice of bread. Top with salmon and arugula.

Top with remaining slice of bread. Enjoy.

Dinner:

Quinoa Bowl with Roasted Vegetables:

Ingredients:

-1 cup quinoa

-2 cups vegetable broth

-1 cup diced sweet potato

-1/2 cup red bell pepper, diced

-1/2 cup yellow bell pepper, diced

-1/2 cup red onion, diced

-1 tablespoon olive oil

-1/4 teaspoon garlic powder

-1/4 teaspoon black pepper

-1/4 teaspoon salt

-1/4 cup crumbled feta cheese

-2 tablespoons balsamic vinegar

Instructions:

Preheat oven to 400 degrees F. Line a baking sheet with parchment paper.

In a medium bowl, combine sweet potato, bell peppers, red onion, olive oil, garlic powder, black pepper, and salt.

Spread mixture on the prepared baking sheet and roast for 20-25 minutes, stirring halfway through. Meanwhile, bring vegetable broth to a boil.

Add quinoa, reduce heat to low, cover, and simmer for 15-20 minutes, or until quinoa is cooked through. In a large bowl, combine roasted vegetables and quinoa. Top with feta cheese and balsamic vinegar. Serve.

Day 3
Breakfast:

Banana Oat Smoothie:

Ingredients:

-1 banana, frozen

-1/2 cup rolled oats

-1/2 cup almond milk

-1/2 teaspoon ground cinnamon

-1/4 teaspoon vanilla extract

Instructions:

In a blender, combine banana, oats, almond milk, cinnamon, and vanilla extract. Blend until smooth. Enjoy.

Lunch:

Lentil Soup:

Ingredients:

-1 tablespoon olive oil

-1 onion, diced

-2 cloves garlic, minced

-1 teaspoon ground cumin

- 1 teaspoon ground coriander

- 1/2 teaspoon dried oregano

- 1/4 teaspoon black pepper-1/4 teaspoon salt

- 2 cups vegetable broth

- 1 cup dried lentils

- 1 can diced tomatoes

- 1 cup spinach, chopped

Instructions:

Warm the olive oil in a big saucepan over medium heat. Add onion and garlic and cook until the onion is tender and transparent.

Add cumin, coriander, oregano, black pepper, and salt. Stir to combine. Add vegetable broth, lentils, and tomatoes. Bring to a boil, reduce heat to low, and simmer for 20-25 minutes, or until lentils are tender. Add spinach and cook for an additional 5 minutes. Serve.

Dinner:

Baked Sweet Potato Fries:

Ingredients:

-2 sweet potatoes, cut into wedges

-2 tablespoons olive oil

-1/4 teaspoon garlic powder

-1/4 teaspoon black pepper-1/4 teaspoon salt

Instructions:

Preheat oven to 425 degrees F. Line a baking sheet with parchment paper.

In a medium bowl, combine sweet potato wedges, olive oil, garlic powder, black pepper, and salt. Spread mixture on the prepared baking sheet and bake for 15-20 minutes, or until fries are crispy. Serve.

Day 4

Breakfast:

Banana-Coconut Smoothie Bowl:

Ingredients:

-1 banana, frozen

-1/2 cup coconut milk

-1/2 cup plain Greek yogurt

-1 teaspoon chia seeds

-1 teaspoon honey

-1/4 cup shredded coconut

Instructions:

In a blender, combine banana, coconut milk, yogurt, chia seeds, and honey.

Blend until smooth. Transfer to a bowl and top with shredded coconut. Enjoy.

Lunch:

Mediterranean Chickpea Salad:

Ingredients:

-1 can chickpeas, drained and rinsed

-1/2 cup cucumber, diced

-1/2 cup red bell pepper, diced

-1/2 cup cherry tomatoes, halved

-1/4 cup red onion, diced

-1 tablespoon olive oil

-1 teaspoon lemon juice

-1/4 teaspoon garlic powder

-1/4 teaspoon black pepper

-1/4 teaspoon salt

-1/4 cup crumbled feta cheese

-1/4 cup chopped fresh parsley

Instructions:

In a large bowl, combine chickpeas, cucumber, bell pepper, cherry tomatoes, and red onion.

In a small bowl, whisk together olive oil, lemon juice, garlic powder, black pepper, and salt. Toss the salad with the dressing to mix. Serve with feta cheese and parsley on top. Serve.

Dinner:

Grilled Portobello Mushrooms:

Ingredients:

-4 portobello mushrooms

-2 tablespoons olive oil

-1 teaspoon balsamic vinegar

-1/4 teaspoon garlic powder

-1/4 teaspoon black pepper

-1/4 teaspoon salt

Instructions:

Preheat a grill to medium-high heat. In a small bowl, whisk together olive oil, balsamic vinegar, garlic powder, black pepper, and salt.

Brush mushrooms with the mixture. Grill mushrooms for 5-7 minutes, or until tender. Serve.

Day 5
Breakfast:

Almond-Coconut Chia Pudding:

Ingredients:

-1/2 cup chia seeds

-1 cup almond milk

-2 tablespoons honey

-1/4 teaspoon vanilla extract

-1/4 cup shredded coconut

-1/4 cup sliced almonds

Instructions:

In a medium bowl, combine chia seeds, almond milk, honey, and vanilla extract. Place the bowl in the refrigerator overnight. In the morning, top with shredded coconut and sliced almonds. Enjoy.

Lunch:

Grilled Cheese Sandwich:

Ingredients:

-2 slices whole-wheat bread

-2 slices cheddar cheese

-2 teaspoons butter

Instructions:

Heat a skillet over medium heat. On one side of each piece of bread, spread butter. Place one slice of bread butter-side down in the skillet.

Top with cheese and remaining slice of bread, butter-side up. Cook for 4-5 minutes, flipping once, or until cheese is melted and bread is golden brown. Serve.

Dinner:

Quinoa-Stuffed Peppers:

Ingredients:

-4 bell peppers, halved and seeds removed

-1 tablespoon olive oil

-1 onion, diced

-2 cloves garlic, minced

-1 teaspoon ground cumin

-1 teaspoon ground coriander

-1/4 teaspoon black pepper

-1/4 teaspoon salt

-1 cup cooked quinoa

-1 can black beans, drained and rinsed

-1 cup corn

-1/2 cup shredded cheddar cheese

Instructions:

Preheat oven to 400 degrees F. Line a baking sheet with parchment paper. Place bell pepper halves on the prepared baking sheet, warm the olive oil in a large pan over medium heat.

Cook until the onion is tender and transparent, about 5 minutes. Add cumin, coriander, black pepper, and salt. Stir to combine.

Add quinoa, black beans, and corn. Stir to combine. Spoon mixture into bell pepper halves.

Top with shredded cheese. Bake the peppers for 25-30 minutes, or until tender. Serve.

Day 6

Breakfast:

Coconut-Pineapple Smoothie:

Ingredients:

-1 banana, frozen

-1/2 cup pineapple, diced

-1/2 cup coconut milk

-1/2 cup plain Greek yogurt

-1/4 cup shredded coconut

Instructions:

In a blender, combine banana, pineapple, coconut milk, yogurt, and shredded coconut. Blend until smooth. Enjoy.

Lunch:

Egg Salad Sandwich:

Ingredients:

-4 eggs, boiled and chopped

-2 tablespoons mayonnaise

-1 teaspoon mustard

-1/4 teaspoon garlic powder

-1/4 teaspoon black pepper

-1/4 teaspoon salt

-2 slices whole-wheat bread

-1/4 cup arugula

Instructions:

In a small bowl, combine eggs, mayonnaise, mustard, garlic powder, black pepper, and salt. On one piece of bread, spread egg salad. Top with arugula and remaining slice of bread. Enjoy.

Dinner:

Baked Tilapia with Garlic-Lemon Sauce:

Ingredients:

-4 tilapia fillets

-2 tablespoons olive oil

-1/4 teaspoon garlic powder

-1/4 teaspoon black pepper

-1/4 teaspoon salt

-1/4 cup white wine

-3 tablespoons lemon juice

-2 tablespoons butter

Instructions:

Preheat oven to 375 degrees F. Line a baking sheet with parchment paper. Place tilapia fillets on the prepared baking sheet and brush with olive oil.

Season with garlic powder, black pepper, and salt. Roast for 15-20 minutes, or until tilapia is cooked through. Meanwhile, in a small saucepan over medium heat, combine white wine, lemon juice, and butter. Cook for 3-4 minutes, or until the sauce thickens. Serve tilapia with garlic-lemon sauce.

Day 7
Breakfast:

Oatmeal-Almond Pancakes:

Ingredients:

- 1/2 cup rolled oats

- 1/2 cup almond milk

- 1 teaspoon baking powder

- 1/4 teaspoon ground cinnamon

- 1/4 teaspoon salt

- 2 tablespoons honey

- 2 tablespoons almond butter

- 1 egg

Instructions:

In a medium bowl, combine oats, almond milk, baking powder, cinnamon, and salt.

In a small bowl, whisk together honey, almond butter, and egg. Pour wet ingredients into the dry ingredients and stir to combine.

Heat a skillet over medium heat. Grease with butter or cooking spray.

Drop batter by the tablespoonful onto the skillet and cook for 2-3 minutes, or until bubbles form.

Flip and cook for an additional 2 minutes, or until golden brown. Serve.

Lunch:

Chickpea and Avocado Wrap:

Ingredients:

-1/2 avocado, mashed

-1 tablespoon olive oil

-1 teaspoon lemon juice

-1/4 teaspoon garlic powder

-1/4 teaspoon black pepper

-1/4 teaspoon salt

-1/2 cup cooked chickpeas

-1/4 cup diced red onion

-1/4 cup diced red bell pepper

-1/4 cup diced cucumber

-1 whole-wheat wrap

-1/4 cup arugula

Instructions:

In a small bowl, whisk together mashed avocado, olive oil, lemon juice, garlic powder, black pepper, and salt.

Spread mixture on the wrap. Top with chickpeas, red onion, red bell pepper, cucumber, and arugula. Roll up wrap and enjoy.

Dinner:

Baked Sweet Potatoes with Avocado-Cilantro Cream:

Ingredients:

-2 sweet potatoes, cut into cubes

-2 tablespoons olive oil

-1/4 teaspoon garlic powder

-1/4 teaspoon black pepper

-1/4 teaspoon salt

-1/2 avocado, mashed

-1 tablespoon lime juice

-1/4 cup fresh cilantro, chopped

-1/4 cup plain Greek yogurt

Instructions:

Preheat oven to 400 degrees F. Line a baking sheet with parchment paper.

In a medium bowl, combine sweet potato cubes, olive oil, garlic powder, black pepper, and salt.

Spread mixture on the prepared baking sheet and roast for 20-25 minutes, stirring halfway through.

Meanwhile, in a small bowl, combine mashed avocado, lime juice, cilantro, and yogurt. Stir to combine. Serve sweet potatoes with avocado-cilantro cream.

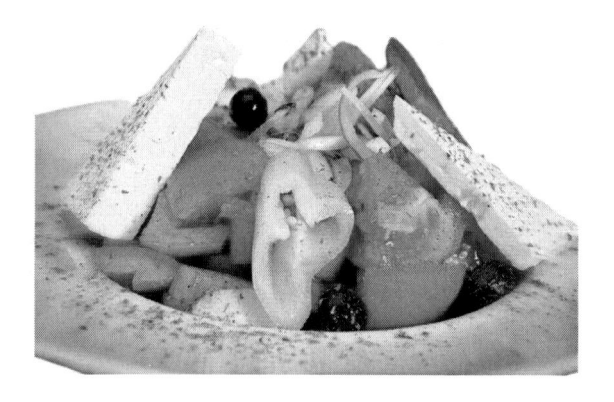

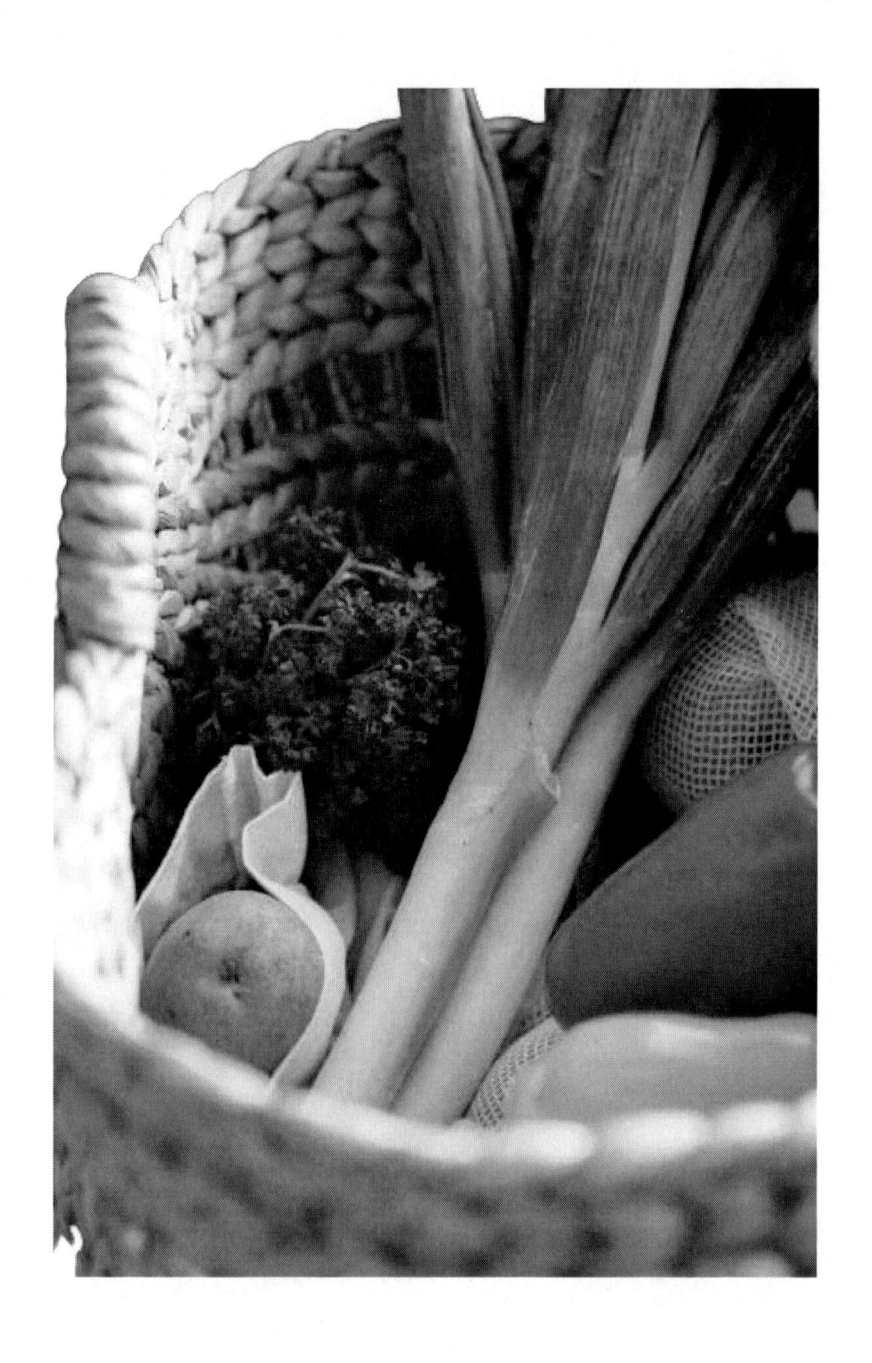

CHAPTER THREE

Sjogren's Syndrome Recipes

BREAKFAST

1. Banana Pancakes with Honey

Ingredients:

2 ripe bananas

2 eggs

¼ teaspoon of baking powder

1 tablespoon of honey

Instructions:

Mash the bananas with a fork in a medium bowl. Beat the eggs and add to the bowl with the banana, stirring to combine.

Add the baking powder and honey and mix until all ingredients are incorporated. Heat a non-stick pan over medium heat.

Drop a spoonful of the batter onto the pan and cook for 2 minutes, flipping once, until both sides are golden brown.

Cooking Time: 15 minutes

2. Yogurt Parfait with Berries

Ingredients:

1 cup of Greek yogurt

¼ cup of granola

1 cup of strawberries

1 cup of blueberries

Instructions:

Place the yogurt in a large bowl. Add the granola and berries and mix together. Layer the parfait into glasses, alternating between the yogurt, granola and berries. Serve cold.

Cooking Time: 10 minutes

3. Avocado Toast with Eggs

Ingredients:

2 slices of whole grain bread

1 avocado

2 eggs,

2 teaspoons of olive oil

Instructions:

Toast the bread in a toaster. In a small pan, heat the olive oil over medium heat. Crack the eggs into the pan and cook until the whites are completely set.

Meanwhile, mash the avocado in a bowl until it is creamy. Spread the mashed avocado over the toasted bread.

Top with the fried eggs and season with salt and pepper to taste.

Cooking Time: 10 minutes

4. Oatmeal with Nuts and Dates

Ingredients:

1 cup of rolled oats

1 teaspoon of cinnamon

1 cup of almond milk

½ cup of sliced almonds

½ cup of chopped dates

Instructions:

In a medium saucepan, combine the oats, cinnamon, almond milk and a pinch of salt.

Bring to a boil and reduce the heat to low. Simmer for 5 minutes, stirring occasionally. Remove from heat and stir in the almonds and dates. Serve warm.

Cooking Time: 10 minutes

5. Poached Pears with Ricotta

Ingredients:

2 pears

2 cups of water

1 teaspoon of honey

½ cup of ricotta cheese

Instructions:

Peel and halve the pears. In a medium pot, bring the water to a boil and add the pears. Simmer for 8 minutes, until the pears are tender.

Remove the pears from the pot and set aside. In a small bowl, mix together the ricotta and honey. Serve the pears warm with the ricotta mixture.

Cooking Time: 10 minutes

6. Egg and Cheese Sandwich

Ingredients:

2 whole wheat English muffins

2 eggs, 2 slices of cheddar cheese

1 tablespoon of butter

Instructions:

Heat a non-stick pan over medium heat. Melt the butter in the pan and add the eggs.

Cook for 3 minutes, flipping once, until the whites are completely set. Meanwhile, toast the English muffins.

Place a slice of cheese on each muffin and top with the cooked eggs. Serve warm.

Cooking Time: 10 minutes

7. Smoothie Bowl with Berries

Ingredients:

1 banana

½ cup of frozen berries

1 cup of almond milk

¼ cup of granola

Instructions:

Place the banana, frozen berries and almond milk in a blender and blend until smooth. Pour the smoothie into a bowl and top with the granola. Serve cold.

Cooking Time: 5 minutes

8. Omelette with Spinach

Ingredients:

2 eggs

2 tablespoons of milk

¼ cup of spinach

1 tablespoon of butter

Instructions:

In a medium bowl, whisk together the eggs and milk. Heat a non-stick pan over medium heat.

Melt the butter in the pan and add the egg mixture. Cook for 3 minutes, stirring occasionally, until the eggs are set.

Add the spinach and cook for an additional 2 minutes. Serve warm.

Cooking Time: 10 minutes

9. Greek Yogurt with Nuts and Honey

Ingredients:

1 cup of Greek yogurt

½ cup of walnuts

1 tablespoon of honey

Instructions:

Place the yogurt in a bowl and top with the walnuts. Drizzle with the honey and stir to combine. Serve cold.

Cooking Time: 5 minutes.

10. Fruit and Nut Granola Bars

Ingredients:

2 cups of rolled oats

¼ cup of honey

1 cup of chopped nuts

1 cup of dried fruit

Instructions:

Preheat the oven to 350°F. In a large bowl, mix together the oats, honey, nuts and dried fruit. Spread the mixture into a parchment-lined baking dish and press down firmly.

Bake for 20 minutes, until golden brown. Cut into bars and serve.

Cooking Time: 30 minutes

11. Salmon and Asparagus with Garlic Lemon Sauce

Ingredients:

- 2 tablespoons extra-virgin olive oil

- 2 cloves garlic, minced

- 2 tablespoons freshly squeezed lemon juice
- 2 tablespoons chopped fresh parsley
- 1/4 teaspoon salt
- 1/4 teaspoon freshly ground black pepper
- 2 (6-ounce) salmon fillets
- 2 cups asparagus, trimmed and cut into 1-inch pieces

Instructions:

1. Preheat the oven to 350°F.

2. Whisk together the olive oil, garlic, lemon juice, parsley, salt, and pepper in a small bowl.

3. Place the salmon fillets and asparagus in a baking dish. Pour the lemon garlic sauce over the top and toss to coat.

4. Bake for 25 to 30 minutes, or until the salmon is cooked through and the asparagus is tender.

5. Serve warm.

12. Vegetable and Quinoa Stew

Ingredients:

- 1 tablespoon olive oil
- 1 onion, diced
- 2 cloves garlic, minced
- 1 red pepper, diced
- 1 zucchini, diced
- 1 tablespoon tomato paste
- 1 teaspoon dried oregano
- 1 teaspoon dried thyme
- 1/2 teaspoon salt
- 1/4 teaspoon freshly ground black pepper
- 2 cups vegetable broth
- 1 (15-ounce) can diced tomatoes
- 1 cup quinoa, rinsed
- 1 (15-ounce) can black beans, rinsed and drained
- 1 cup frozen corn

Instructions:

1. In a large pot over medium heat, heat the olive oil.

2. Add the onion, garlic, red pepper, and zucchini and cook for 5 minutes, or until the vegetables are softened.

3. Stir in the tomato paste, oregano, thyme, salt, and pepper and cook for 1 minute.

4. Add the vegetable broth, diced tomatoes, quinoa, black beans, and corn and bring to a boil.

5. Reduce the heat to low and simmer for 25 minutes, or until the quinoa is cooked through.

6. Serve warm.

13. Creamy Cauliflower Soup
Ingredients:

- 1 tablespoon olive oil

- 1 onion, diced

- 2 cloves garlic, minced

- 2 heads cauliflower, cut into florets

- 2 cups vegetable broth

- 1/2 teaspoon salt

- 1/4 teaspoon freshly ground black pepper

- 1 cup plain Greek yogurt

- 2 tablespoons chopped fresh parsley

Instructions:

1. In a large pot over medium heat, heat the olive oil.

2. Add the onion and garlic and cook for 5 minutes, or until the vegetables are softened.

3. Add the cauliflower, vegetable broth, salt, and pepper and bring to a boil.

4. Reduce the heat to low and simmer for 15 minutes, or until the cauliflower is tender.

5. Place the soup in a blender and puree until smooth.

6. Return the soup to the pot and stir in the Greek yogurt.

7. Heat the soup until warmed through.

8. Serve warm, garnished with parsley.

14. Avocado and Tomato Quinoa Salad

Ingredients:

- 2 cups quinoa, rinsed

- 2 cups water

- 1/2 teaspoon salt

- 1 ripe avocado, diced

- 2 Roma tomatoes, diced

- 1/4 cup freshly squeezed lime juice

- 2 tablespoons extra-virgin olive oil

- 1/4 teaspoon freshly ground black pepper

- 2 tablespoons chopped fresh cilantro

Instructions:

1. Combine the quinoa, water, and salt in a medium saucepan. Bring to a boil, then reduce the heat to low and simmer for 15 minutes, or until the quinoa is cooked through.

2. Transfer the quinoa to a large bowl and add the avocado, tomatoes, lime juice, olive oil, and pepper. Toss to combine.

3. Serve the salad warm or chilled, garnished with cilantro.

15. Baked Cod with Spinach and Tomatoes

Ingredients:

• 2 tablespoons olive oil

• 2 cloves garlic, minced

• 1 teaspoon dried oregano

• 1/2 teaspoon salt

• 1/4 teaspoon freshly ground black pepper

• 2 (6-ounce) cod fillets

• 1 (10-ounce) package frozen spinach, thawed and squeezed dry

• 2 Roma tomatoes, diced

• 2 tablespoons freshly squeezed lemon juice

Instructions:

1. Preheat the oven to 350°F.

2. In a small bowl, whisk together the olive oil, garlic, oregano, salt, and pepper.

3. Arrange the cod fillets in a baking pan. Pour the olive oil mixture over the top and spread the spinach and tomatoes on top.

4. Bake for 25 minutes, or until the cod is cooked through.

5. Drizzle the lemon juice over the top and serve warm.

16. No-Bake Oatmeal Cookies

Ingredients:

- 2 cups old-fashioned rolled oats

- 1/2 cup creamy almond butter

- 1/2 cup honey

- 1 teaspoon vanilla extract

- 1/4 teaspoon salt

- 1/2 cup finely chopped pecans

- 1/2 cup dried cranberries

Instructions:

1. In a large bowl, combine the oats, almond butter, honey, vanilla extract, and salt. Stir until well combined.

2. Stir in the pecans and dried cranberries.

3. Lay parchment paper on a baking sheet.

4. Using your hands, shape the mixture into 1-inch balls and place on the baking sheet.

5. Place the baking sheet in the refrigerator for 20 minutes.

6. Serve chilled.

17. Zucchini and Carrot Fritters

Ingredients:

- 1 cup grated zucchini

- 1 cup grated carrot

- 1/2 cup all-purpose flour

- 1/2 teaspoon baking powder

- 1/2 teaspoon salt

- 1/4 teaspoon freshly ground black pepper

- 2 eggs, lightly beaten

- 2 tablespoons olive oil

Instructions:

1. In a large bowl, combine the zucchini, carrot, flour, baking powder, salt, and pepper. Stir until well combined.

2. Stir in the eggs until well combined.

3. In a large skillet over medium heat, heat the olive oil.

4. Drop the batter by heaping tablespoons into the skillet and flatten with a spatula.

5. Cook each side for 3 to 4 minutes, or until golden brown.

6. Transfer to a plate lined with paper towels.

7. Serve warm.

18. Baked Sweet Potato Fries

Ingredients:

- 4 sweet potatoes, peeled and cut into fries

- 2 tablespoons olive oil

- 1/2 teaspoon salt

- 1/4 teaspoon freshly ground black pepper

- 1/4 teaspoon garlic powder

Instructions:

1. Preheat the oven to 425°F.

2. Lay parchment paper on a baking sheet.

3. In a large bowl, combine the sweet potatoes, olive oil, salt, pepper, and garlic powder. Toss to coat.

4. Spread the sweet potatoes in an even layer on the baking sheet.

5. Bake for 20 minutes, flip the fries, and bake for an additional 20 minutes, or until golden brown and crispy.

6. Serve warm

19. Baked Eggplant Parmesan

Ingredients:

- 2 eggplants, sliced into 1/4-inch-thick slices

- 2 tablespoons olive oil

- 1/2 teaspoon salt
- 1/4 teaspoon freshly ground black pepper
- 1 cup marinara sauce
- 1 cup shredded mozzarella cheese
- 1/4 cup freshly grated Parmesan cheese
- 2 tablespoons chopped fresh basil

Instructions:

1. Preheat the oven to 375°F.

2. Lay parchment paper on a baking sheet.

3. In a large bowl, combine the eggplant slices, olive oil, salt, and pepper. Toss to coat.

4. Place the eggplant slices on the baking sheet and bake for 15 minutes, or until golden brown.

5. Remove from the oven and spread the marinara sauce over the top.

6. Sprinkle the mozzarella cheese, Parmesan cheese, and basil over the top.

7. Bake for an additional 15 minutes, or until the cheese is melted and bubbly.

8. Serve warm.

20. Banana Oat Smoothie

Ingredients:

- 1 banana, peeled and frozen
- 1 cup unsweetened almond milk
- 1/2 cup rolled oats
- 1 teaspoon honey
- 1/4 teaspoon ground cinnamon

Instructions:

1. In a blender, combine all of the ingredients and blend until smooth.

2. Serve immediately.

LUNCH

1. Salmon and Avocado Wraps

Ingredients:

- 4 ounces of salmon, cooked
- 1/2 ripe avocado, diced
- 2 tablespoons of light mayonnaise
- 2 tablespoons of minced red onion
- 2 large whole-wheat tortillas
- Salt and pepper, to taste

Instruction:

1. In a medium bowl, combine the salmon, avocado, mayonnaise, and red onion.

2. Season with salt and pepper, to taste.

3. Place the tortillas on a flat work surface.

4. Spread the salmon mixture evenly over each tortilla.

5. Roll up the tortillas and cut them in half.

6. Serve immediately.

2. Quinoa and Vegetable Bowl

Ingredients:

- 1 cup of quinoa, cooked
- 1 cup of diced bell peppers
- 1/4 cup of diced red onion
- 1/4 cup of diced carrots
- 1/4 cup of diced celery
- 2 tablespoons of olive oil
- Salt and pepper, to taste

Instructions:

1. Preheat the oven to 375°F.

2. In a medium bowl, combine the quinoa, bell peppers, red onion, carrots, and celery.

3. Drizzle with the olive oil and season with salt and pepper, to taste.

4. Distribute the mixture on a baking sheet.

5. Bake for 25 minutes, stirring occasionally.

6. Serve warm.

3. Sesame Chicken Salad

Ingredients:

- 4 ounces of cooked chicken, diced

- 1/2 cup of diced cucumber

- 1/4 cup of diced bell pepper

- 1/4 cup of diced red onion

- 2 tablespoons of sesame oil

- 2 tablespoons of rice vinegar

- 2 tablespoons of toasted sesame seeds

- Salt and pepper, to taste

Instructions:

1. In a medium bowl, combine the chicken, cucumber, bell pepper, and red onion.

2. Drizzle with the sesame oil and rice vinegar.

3. Sprinkle with the sesame seeds and season with salt and pepper, to taste.

4. Toss to combine.

5. Serve chilled.

4. Salmon and Broccoli Bowl

Ingredients:

- 4 ounces of salmon, cooked

- 1 cup of cooked broccoli florets

- 2 tablespoons of olive oil

- 2 tablespoons of lemon juice

- 2 tablespoons of minced garlic

- Salt and pepper, to taste

Instructions:

1. Preheat the oven to 375°F.

2. In a medium bowl, combine the salmon and broccoli.

3. Drizzle with the lemon juice and olive oil.

4. Sprinkle with the garlic and season with salt and pepper, to taste.

5. Distribute the mixture on a baking sheet.

6. Bake for 30 minutes, stirring occasionally.

7. Serve warm.

5. Zucchini and Tomato Salad

Ingredients:

- 1/2 cup of diced zucchini
- 1/2 cup of diced tomatoes
- 2 tablespoons of olive oil
- 2 tablespoons of balsamic vinegar
- 2 tablespoons of minced fresh basil
- Salt and pepper, to taste

Instructions:

1. In a medium bowl, combine the zucchini and tomatoes.

2. Drizzle the olive oil and balsamic vinegar over the top.

3. Sprinkle with the basil and season with salt and pepper, to taste.

4. Toss to combine.

5. Serve chilled

6. Sweet Potato and Bean Burrito

Ingredients:

- 1/2 cup of cooked sweet potatoes, mashed
- 1/2 cup of cooked black beans
- 2 tablespoons of minced red onion
- 2 teaspoons of chili powder
- 2 large whole-wheat tortillas
- Salt and pepper, to taste

Instructions:

1. Preheat the oven to 375°F.

2. In a medium bowl, combine the sweet potatoes, black beans, red onion, and chili powder.

3. Season to taste with salt and pepper.

4. Place the tortillas on a flat work surface.

5. Spread the sweet potato mixture evenly over each tortilla.

6. Roll up the tortillas and place them on a baking sheet.

7. Bake for 25 minutes.

8. Serve warm.

7. Avocado and Egg Salad

Ingredients:

- 2 hard-boiled eggs, diced
- 1/2 ripe avocado, diced
- 2 tablespoons of light mayonnaise
- 2 tablespoons of minced red onion
- 2 teaspoons of freshly squeezed lemon juice
- Salt and pepper, to taste

Instructions:

1. In a medium bowl, combine the eggs, avocado, mayonnaise, red onion, and lemon juice.

2. Season with salt and pepper, to taste.

3. Toss to combine.

4. Serve chilled.

8. Grilled Vegetable Wrap

Ingredients:

- 1/2 cup of diced bell peppers
- 1/4 cup of diced red onion
- 2 tablespoons of olive oil
- 2 large whole-wheat tortillas
- Salt and pepper, to taste

Instructions:

1. Preheat the oven to 375°F.

2. In a medium bowl, combine the bell peppers and red onion.

3. Drizzle with the olive oil and season with salt and pepper, to taste.

4. Spread the mixture evenly onto a baking sheet.

5. Bake for 20 minutes, stirring occasionally.

6. Place the tortillas on a flat work surface.

7. Spread the grilled vegetables evenly over each tortilla.

8. Roll up the tortillas and cut them in half.

9. Serve warm.

9. Lentil and Spinach Salad – 20 minutes

Ingredients:

- 1 cup of cooked lentils

- 2 cups of fresh spinach

- 1/4 cup of diced bell pepper

- 2 tablespoons of olive oil

- 2 tablespoons of freshly squeezed lemon juice

- 2 tablespoons of minced fresh parsley

- Salt and pepper, to taste

Instructions:

1. Preheat the oven to 375°F.

2. In a medium bowl, combine the lentils, spinach, and bell pepper.

3. Drizzle with the lemon juice and olive oil.

4. Sprinkle with the parsley and season with salt and pepper, to taste.

5. Transfer the mixture to a baking sheet.

6. Bake for 20 minutes, stirring occasionally.

7. Serve warm.

10. Mushroom and Quinoa Bowl – 25 minutes

Ingredients:

- 1 cup of quinoa, cooked
- 1 cup of diced mushrooms
- 2 tablespoons of olive oil
- 2 tablespoons of balsamic vinegar
- 2 tablespoons of minced fresh parsley
- Salt and pepper, to taste

Instructions:

1. Preheat the oven to 375°F.

2. In a medium bowl, combine the quinoa and mushrooms.

3. Drizzle with the olive oil and balsamic vinegar.

4. Sprinkle with the parsley and season with salt and pepper, to taste.

5. Spread the mixture onto a baking sheet.

6. Bake for 25 minutes, stirring occasionally.

7. Serve warm.

DINNER

1. Spanish-Style Stuffed Peppers

Ingredients:

-4 bell peppers

-1/2 cup cooked quinoa

-1/2 cup canned black beans

-1/2 cup cooked corn

-1/2 cup diced onions

-1/4 cup diced tomatoes

-1/4 cup diced green chilies

-1 garlic clove, minced

-1 teaspoon cumin

-1 teaspoon chili powder

-1/2 teaspoon dried oregano

-1/2 teaspoon paprika

-Salt and pepper to taste

-1/4 cup reduced-fat shredded cheese

Instructions:

1. Preheat oven to 350°F.

2. Cut the tops off the peppers and hollow out the insides.

3. In a large bowl, combine the quinoa, black beans, corn, onions, tomatoes, green chilies, garlic, cumin, chili powder, oregano, paprika, salt and pepper. Mix until everything is combined.

4. Fill the peppers with the quinoa mixture and sprinkle the cheese over the top.

5. Place the peppers in a baking dish and bake for 25 minutes, or until the peppers are tender and the cheese is melted.

Cooking Time: 25 minutes

2. Baked Salmon with Roasted Vegetables

Ingredients:

-4 salmon fillets

-1/2 cup diced zucchini

-1/2 cup diced yellow squash

-1/2 cup diced red bell pepper

-1/4 cup diced onion

-2 tablespoons olive oil

-2 tablespoons lemon juice

-1 teaspoon garlic powder

-Salt and pepper to taste

Instructions:

1. Preheat oven to 400°F.

2. In a large bowl, combine the zucchini, squash, bell pepper, and onion.

Drizzle with the olive oil, lemon juice, garlic powder, salt and pepper.

Mix until everything is well coated.

3. Place the salmon fillets in a baking dish and top with the roasted vegetables.

4. Bake for 20 minutes, or until the salmon is cooked through and the vegetables are tender.

Cooking Time: 20 minutes

3. Quinoa Bowl with Turkey and Veggies

Ingredients:

-1/2 cup cooked quinoa

-4 ounces cooked turkey, diced

-1/2 cup diced carrots

-1/2 cup diced zucchini

-1/4 cup diced onion

-2 tablespoons olive oil

-1 tablespoon balsamic vinegar

-1 teaspoon minced garlic

-Salt and pepper to taste

Instructions:

1. Preheat oven to 400°F.

2. In a large bowl, combine the quinoa, turkey, carrots, zucchini, and onion.

Drizzle with the olive oil, balsamic vinegar, garlic, salt and pepper. Mix until everything is well coated.

3. Spread the quinoa mixture onto a baking sheet and bake for 15 minutes, or until the vegetables are tender.

Cooking Time: 15 minutes

4. Slow Cooker Chicken and Quinoa Stew

Ingredients:

-1-pound boneless, skinless chicken breasts

-1 cup cooked quinoa

-1 can diced tomatoes

-1/2 cup diced carrots

-1/2 cup diced celery

-1/2 cup diced onion

-1 teaspoon garlic powder

-1 teaspoon dried oregano

-Salt and pepper to taste

Instructions:

1. Place the chicken, quinoa, tomatoes, carrots, celery, onion, garlic powder, oregano, salt and pepper in a slow cooker.

2. Cover and cook on low for 6-8 hours, or until the chicken is cooked through and the vegetables are tender.

Cooking Time: 6-8 hours

5. Sautéed Shrimp and Veggies

Ingredients:

-1 pound peeled and deveined shrimp

- 1/2 cup diced red bell pepper

- 1/2 cup diced zucchini

- 1/2 cup diced mushrooms

- 1/4 cup diced onion

- 2 tablespoons olive oil

- 1 tablespoon minced garlic

- 1 tablespoon fresh lemon juice

- Salt and pepper to taste

Instructions:

1. Heat the olive oil in a large skillet over medium heat.

2. Add the shrimp, bell pepper, zucchini, mushrooms, and onion. Sauté for 5 minutes, or until the vegetables are tender.

3. Add the garlic, lemon juice, salt and pepper. Sauté for 2 minutes more.

Cooking Time: 7 minutes

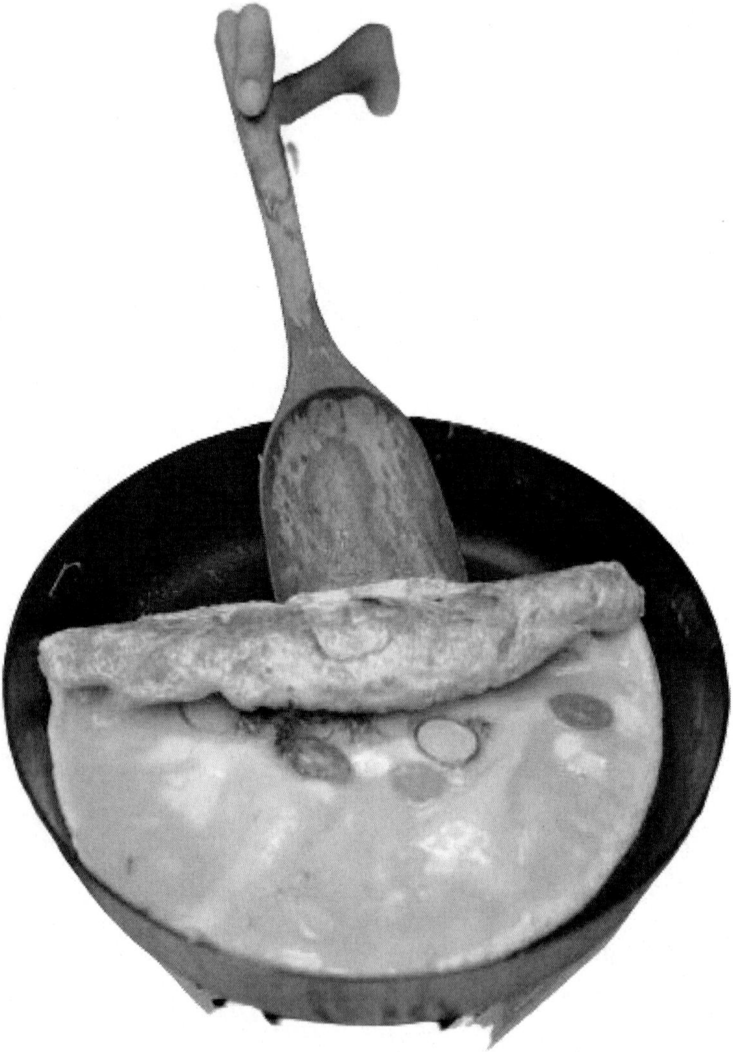

CONCLUSION

Sjogren's syndrome is an autoimmune disorder that affects the moisture-producing glands in the body, leading to dryness in the eyes, mouth, and other mucous membranes.

It is important that people with Sjogren's syndrome follow a healthy diet to help manage symptoms and reduce the risk of complications.

A well-balanced diet should focus on eating plenty of fruits, vegetables, and whole grains. It is critical to limit processed foods and foods high in saturated fat and sugar.

Additionally, foods high in omega-3 fatty acids, such as fatty fish, nuts, and seeds, are beneficial for people with Sjogren's syndrome because they help reduce inflammation.

Adequate hydration is also important for people with Sjogren's syndrome since dryness is a major symptom.

Drinking enough fluids can help keep mucous membranes moist and reduce discomfort.

Additionally, avoiding alcohol and caffeine may help reduce dryness.

In conclusion, having Sjogren's syndrome does not mean that you have to give up your favourite foods or stop eating out.

However, it is important to be mindful of what you eat and drink in order to manage symptoms and reduce the risk of complications.

Eating a well-balanced diet, limiting processed foods, and drinking plenty of fluids can help manage Sjogren's syndrome and improve overall health.

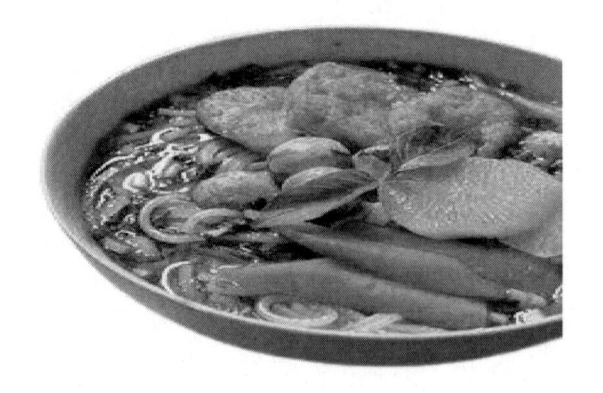

Manufactured by Amazon.ca
Acheson, AB